THE PREGNANCY
Anti-Inflammatory Diet

Copyright

The Pregnancy Anti-Inflammatory Diet: 80 Delicious Recipes for a Healthy Pregnancy

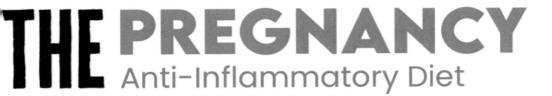

THE PREGNANCY
Anti-Inflammatory Diet

80 DELICIOUS RECIPES FOR A HEALTHY PREGNANCY

RACHEL MORGAN

Disclaimer

The information provided in "The Pregnancy Anti-Inflammatory Diet: 80 Delicious Recipes for a Healthy Pregnancy" is for educational purposes only and is not intended as a substitute for professional medical advice or treatment. Always seek the advice of your healthcare provider before making any changes to your diet or lifestyle during pregnancy.

The author and publisher of this book are not healthcare professionals, and the content of this book should not be considered as medical advice. The recipes and dietary recommendations in this book are based on significant knowledge about anti-inflammatory diets and healthy eating during pregnancy, but every pregnancy is unique, and individual dietary needs may vary. It is essential to consult with your healthcare provider or a qualified medical professional for personalized advice regarding your specific health condition, dietary restrictions, or concerns during pregnancy.

The recipes in this book may include various ingredients that may cause allergies or adverse reactions in some individuals. It is the responsibility of the reader to review the ingredient list, consult with their healthcare provider, and avoid any allergens or ingredients that may pose a risk to their health or the health of their baby.

The author and publisher of this book do not assume any liability or responsibility for any loss, damage, or adverse consequences arising directly or indirectly from the use or application of any information or recipes provided in this book. The reader is solely responsible for their use of the information and recipes in this book and assumes all risks associated with such use.

Please note that the dietary recommendations and guidelines for pregnant women may change over time due to advances in scientific research or updates in medical guidelines. It is recommended to stay informed about the latest research and guidelines from reputable sources and consult with a qualified healthcare provider for the most up-to-date and accurate information.

By using this book, you acknowledge and agree to the above disclaimer and understand that the author and publisher of this book are not liable for any loss or damage resulting from the use of the information or recipes provided in this book. Always consult with your healthcare provider or a qualified medical professional for personalized medical advice during pregnancy.

Dedication

This book is dedicated to all the expecting mothers who are embarking on the beautiful journey of pregnancy. Your strength, resilience, and love are truly awe-inspiring.

To the women who are nurturing a new life within them, this book is for you. May it be a guiding light on your path to a healthy and happy pregnancy.

To the little miracles growing inside, you are already loved beyond measure. This book is dedicated to helping you thrive with the nourishing power of food.

To my family and friends, thank you for your unwavering support and encouragement. Your love has been my driving force in creating this book.

To the amazing team behind this book, your dedication and passion are deeply appreciated. Thank you for helping me bring this vision to life.

And lastly, to my beloved, who has been my rock and my inspiration, thank you for your unwavering belief in me. This book is dedicated to you and our little one, with all my love.

Here's to a journey of health, happiness, and delicious food during pregnancy!

With love,
Rachel Morgan

TABLE OF CONTENTS

ABOUT THE AUTHOR

Rachel Morgan is a nutritionist and wellness expert with a passion for empowering expectant mothers to have healthy and vibrant pregnancies. With years of experience in the field of nutrition and a deep understanding of the unique nutritional needs during pregnancy, Rachel Morgan has helped countless women achieve optimal health and well-being during this special time in their lives.

As a dedicated advocate for maternal health, Rachel Morgan has conducted extensive research on the impact of diet and nutrition on pregnancy outcomes. Through her work, she has discovered the powerful role that an anti-inflammatory diet can play in supporting a healthy pregnancy. Her expertise in this area has led her to write "The Pregnancy Anti-Inflammatory Diet: 80 Delicious Recipes for a Healthy Pregnancy" as a comprehensive guide for expectant mothers who want to prioritize their health and the health of their babies during pregnancy.

One of the highlights of "The Pregnancy Anti-Inflammatory Diet" is the collection of 80 delicious and wholesome recipes that Rachel Morgan has carefully crafted to support a healthy pregnancy. These recipes are designed to be easy to prepare, nutrient-dense, and packed with flavor, making them perfect for busy expectant mothers who want to enjoy delicious meals while nourishing their bodies and their growing babies.

With Rachel Morgan's guidance, readers will learn how to make informed food choices, create balanced and satisfying meals, and develop healthy eating habits that will benefit them and their babies throughout pregnancy and beyond. Her compassionate and evidence-based approach to nutrition empowers expectant mothers to take control of their health and make choices that will positively impact their pregnancy journey.

As a leading authority on nutrition for pregnancy, Rachel Morgan is passionate about helping expectant mothers achieve optimal health for themselves and their babies. Her expertise, compassion, and commitment to empowering women make "The Pregnancy Anti-Inflammatory Diet" an indispensable guide for any woman who wants to have a healthy, vibrant, and nourished pregnancy journey.

GREEK YOGURT WITH MIXED BERRIES & CHIA SEEDS

READY IN ABOUT: 5 MIN

READY IN ABOUT: 0 MIN

SERVINGS: 1

Ingredients

- 1 cup Greek yogurt without added sugar
- 1/2 cup mixed berries (e.g., blueberries, raspberries, strawberries)
- 2 tbsp chia seeds
- 1 tbsp honey (optional)

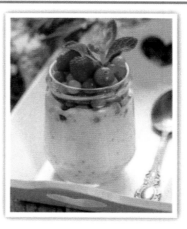

Directions

1. In a bowl, mix the Greek yogurt and honey (if using).
2. Top with mixed berries and chia seeds.
3. Enjoy immediately or refrigerate for up to 2 hours.

AVOCADO TOAST WITH POACHED EGG

READY IN ABOUT: 10 MIN

READY IN ABOUT: 5 MIN

SERVINGS: 1

Ingredients

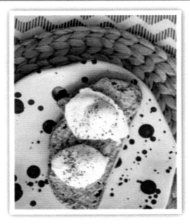

- 1 slice of whole-grain bread
- 1/2 ripe avocado
- 1 egg
- Salt and pepper, to taste
- Red pepper flakes (optional)

Directions

1. Toast bread until crisp. Using a fork, mash the avocado, and then add salt and pepper to taste. Spread mashed avocado on toast.
2. Poach the egg: Fill a saucepan with water, boil, and simmer. Slip the egg into the heating water in a small cup. Remove with a slotted spoon after 3–4 minutes.
3. Season the avocado toast with salt, pepper, and red pepper flakes, then top with the poached egg. Serve right away.

OVERNIGHT OATS WITH FLAXSEEDS AND FRUITS

READY IN ABOUT: 10 MIN

READY IN ABOUT: 0 MIN

SERVINGS: 1

Ingredients

- 1/2 cup rolled oats
- 3/4 cup almond milk
- 1 tbsp flaxseeds
- 1/2 cup mixed fruit (e.g., chopped apples, berries, bananas)
- 1 tbsp honey or maple syrup (optional)

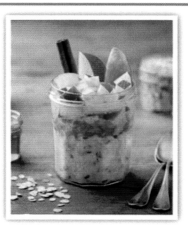

Directions

1. In a jar or bowl, combine the rolled oats, almond milk, flaxseeds, and sweetener (if using).
2. Cover and free overnight or for at least 6 hours.
3. In the morning, top with mixed fruit and enjoy.

SPINACH, MUSHROOM, AND SHRIMP OMELETTE

READY IN ABOUT: 10 MIN

READY IN ABOUT: 10 MIN

SERVINGS: 1

Ingredients

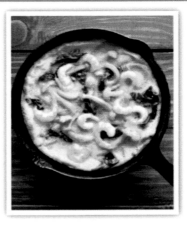

- 2 eggs
- 1/2 cup chopped fresh spinach
- 1/2 cup sliced mushrooms
- 1/4 cup diced onion
- 1/4 cup shredded cheese (optional)
- 1/4 cup cooked shrimp, peeled and chopped
- 1 tbsp olive oil
- Salt and pepper, to taste

Directions

1. Whisk eggs with salt and pepper in a bowl
2. Heat olive oil on medium in a non-stick skillet. Cook onions and mushrooms for 5 minutes until tender.
3. Add the chopped shrimp to the skillet and cook for an additional 2 minutes.
4. Wilt spinach for 1-2 minutes.
5. Tilt the pan to spread the whisked eggs over the vegetables and shrimp. Cook for 3-4 minutes.
6. Sprinkle cheese on half the omelet and fold the other half over it. Cook the cheese for 1 to 2 minutes to melt it.
7. Place the omelet on a plate immediately and serve.

ALMOND BUTTER AND BANANA SMOOTHIE

READY IN ABOUT: 5 MIN

READY IN ABOUT: 0 MIN

SERVINGS: 1

Ingredients

- 1 banana
- 1 cup unsweetened almond milk
- 1 tbsp almond butter
- 1 tbsp chia seeds
- 1/2 cup ice (optional)

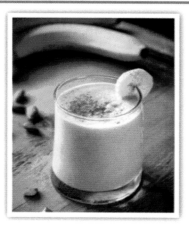

Directions

1. In a food processor, combine the banana, almond milk, almond butter, chia seeds, and ice (if using).
2. Blend until smooth and creamy.
3. Pour into a glass and enjoy immediately.

QUINOA PORRIDGE WITH NUTS AND DRIED FRUITS

READY IN ABOUT: 5 MIN

READY IN ABOUT: 20 MIN

SERVINGS: 2

Ingredients

- 1/2 cup uncooked quinoa
- 1 cup water
- 1 cup almond milk
- 1/4 cup chopped nuts (e.g., almonds, walnuts, pecans)
- 1/4 cup dried fruits (e.g., raisins, cranberries, apricots)
- 1 tbsp honey or maple syrup (optional)
- 1/2 tsp cinnamon

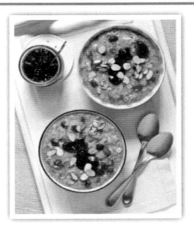

Directions

1. Mix the rice and water in a pot. Take to a boil, reduce heat to low, cover, and simmer for 15 minutes until quinoa is soft and water is absorbed.
2. Mix almond milk, almonds, dried fruits, sugar, and cinnamon. Stir occasionally for 5 more minutes.
3. Put the cereal in two bowls and serve it hot.

CHIA SEED PUDDING WITH FRESH FRUIT

READY IN ABOUT: 5 MIN

READY IN ABOUT: 0 MIN

SERVINGS: 0

Ingredients

- 1/4 cup chia seeds
- 1 cup almond milk
- 1 tbsp honey or maple syrup (optional)
- 1/2 tsp vanilla extract
- 1 cup fresh fruit (e.g., berries, mango, kiwi)

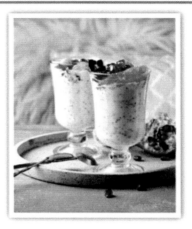

Directions

1. In a jar or bowl, combine the chia seeds, almond milk, sweetener (if using), and vanilla extract.
2. Cover and freeze overnight or for approx 6 hours.
3. When ready to serve, stir the pudding well and divide it between two bowls. Top with fresh fruit, and enjoy.

BUCKWHEAT PANCAKES WITH BLUEBERRIES

READY IN ABOUT: 10 MIN

READY IN ABOUT: 15 MIN

SERVINGS: 4

Ingredients

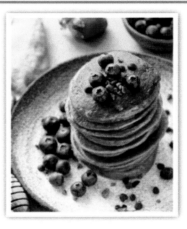

- 1 cup buckwheat flour
- 1 cup almond milk
- 1 egg
- 2 tbsp melted coconut oil or unsalted butter
- 1 tbsp honey or maple syrup
- 1 tsp baking powder
- 1/2 tsp salt
- 1 cup fresh blueberries
- Cooking spray or additional coconut oil for greasing

Directions

1. Mix buckwheat flour, baking powder, and salt in a bowl. Mix almond milk, egg-melted coconut oil, and sweetener
2. in another bowl.
3. Mix the wet and dry components. Mix blueberries gently.
4. Lightly grease a non-stick skillet or griddle over medium heat.
5. Pour 1/4 cup batter per pancake onto the heated surface. Once bubbles appear, rotate and fry for another 2-3 mins until it gets golden brown and cooked through.
6. Serve the pancakes warm with additional blueberries and a drizzle of honey or maple syrup.

KIWI AND BERRY GREEN SMOOTHIE BOWL WITH KALE AND SPIRULINA

READY IN ABOUT: 10 MIN

READY IN ABOUT: 0 MIN

SERVINGS: 1

Ingredients

- 1/2 cup chopped kale
- 1/2 cup frozen berries (e.g., strawberries, blueberries)
- 1 kiwi, peeled and chopped
- 1 tsp spirulina powder
- 1/2 cup unsweetened almond milk
- Toppings: sliced fruit (e.g., kiwi, berries), granola, nuts, coconut flakes, chia seeds

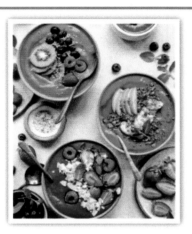

Directions

1. Combine the chopped kale, frozen berries, chopped kiwi, spirulina powder, and almond milk in a blender.
2. Blend until smooth and creamy. If needed, add more almond milk to reach the desired consistency.
3. Pour the smoothie into a serving bowl and add your desired toppings.
4. Enjoy immediately.

WHOLE GRAIN MUESLI WITH ALMOND MILK

READY IN ABOUT: 5 MIN

READY IN ABOUT: 0 MIN

SERVINGS: 2

Ingredients

- 1 cup whole grain muesli (store-bought or homemade)
- 1 cup unsweetened almond milk
- 1/2 cup chopped fresh fruit (e.g., apples, berries)
- 1/4 cup chopped nuts (e.g., almonds, walnuts, pecans)
- 1/4 cup dried fruits (e.g., raisins, cranberries, apricots)
- 1 tbsp honey or maple syrup (optional)

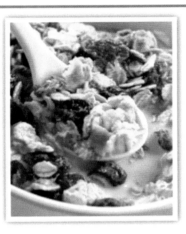

Directions

1. In a bowl, mix the whole-grain muesli with almond milk. Allow it to rest for a few mins to soften.
2. Stir in the chopped fresh fruit, nuts, and dried fruits. Add sweetener if desired.
3. Divide the muesli between two bowls and serve.

VEGGIE EGG SCRAMBLE

READY IN ABOUT: 10 MIN

READY IN ABOUT: 10 MIN

SERVINGS: 1

Ingredients

- 2 eggs
- 1/2 cup chopped bell pepper
- 1/2 cup chopped tomato
- 1/4 cup diced onion
- 1/4 cup shredded cheese (optional)
- 1 tbsp olive oil
- Salt and pepper, to taste

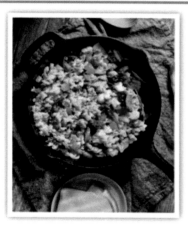

Directions

1. In a bowl, whisk the eggs and season with salt and pepper.
2. In a non-stick skillet, warm the olive oil over moderate heat. Add the onions, bell pepper, and tomato, and cook for 5 minutes or until softened.
3. Pour the whisked eggs over the vegetables, stirring to combine. Cook for 3-4 mins until the eggs are set.
4. Sprinkle cheese (if using) on top and cook for another 1-2 minutes to melt the cheese. Transfer the scramble to a plate and serve immediately.

BERRY ALMOND SMOOTHIE

READY IN ABOUT: 5 MIN

READY IN ABOUT: 0 MIN

SERVINGS: 1

Ingredients

- 1 cup mixed berries (fresh or frozen)
- 1/2 cup unsweetened almond milk
- 1/4 cup Greek yogurt
- 1 tbsp almond butter
- 1 tbsp chia seeds
- 1/2 cup ice (optional)

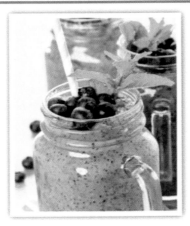

Directions

1. Combine the mixed berries, almond milk, Greek yogurt, almond butter, chia seeds, and ice (if using).
2. Blend until smooth and creamy.
3. Pour into a glass and enjoy immediately.

APPLE CINNAMON OATMEAL

READY IN ABOUT: 5 MIN

READY IN ABOUT: 10 MIN

SERVINGS: 2

Ingredients

- 1 cup rolled oats
- 1 cup water
- 1 cup unsweetened almond milk
- 1 apple, peeled, cored, and chopped
- 2 tbsp honey or maple syrup
- 1/2 tsp cinnamon
- Pinch of salt

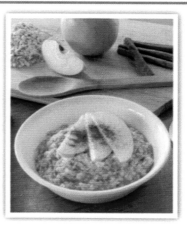

Directions

1. Combine the rolled oats, water, and almond milk in a saucepan. Reduce heat to moderate and simmer for 5 mins while stirring occasionally.
2. Stir in the apple chunks, sugar, cinnamon, and salt. Continue cooking for 5 minutes or until the oats are creamy and the pears are tender. Warm the oatmeal and divide it between two containers.

SWEET POTATO AND SPINACH FRITTATA

READY IN ABOUT: 15 MIN

READY IN ABOUT: 20 MIN

SERVINGS: 4

Ingredients

- 6 eggs
- 1 medium sweet potato, peeled and diced
- 2 cups fresh spinach
- 1/2 cup diced onion
- 1/4 cup crumbled feta cheese (optional)
- 2 tbsp olive oil
- Salt and pepper, to taste

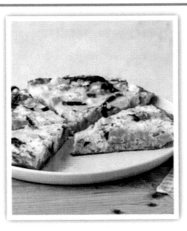

Directions

1. Turn the oven's temperature to 375°F (190°C). Heat olive oil on moderate heat in a large oven-safe skillet. Cook diced sweet potato for 8-10 minutes until tender. Add diced onion and simmer for 3–4 mins.
2. Add the spinach to the pan and prepare for about two to three minutes or until
3. it has softened.
4. Whisk eggs with salt and pepper in a bowl. Spread the eggs evenly over the sautéed vegetables.
5. Sprinkle the feta cheese over the frittata if you want to use it.
6. Prepare the pan in a preheated oven for 12 to 15 minutes or until the frittata is set and the edges are golden brown. Let the frittata cool before slicing and serving.

MANGO AND COCONUT CHIA PUDDING

READY IN ABOUT: 5 MIN

READY IN ABOUT: 0 MIN

SERVINGS: 2

Ingredients

- 1/4 cup chia seeds
- 1 cup coconut milk (without added sugar)
- 1 tbsp honey or maple syrup (optional)
- 1/2 tsp vanilla extract
- 1 cup chopped fresh mango

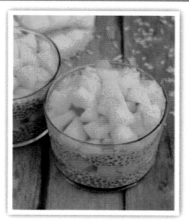

Directions

1. In a jar or bowl, combine the chia seeds, coconut milk, sweetener (if using), and vanilla extract.
2. Cover and freeze overnight or for approx 6 hours.
3. When ready to serve, stir the pudding well and divide it between two bowls. Top with chopped mango, and enjoy.

OAT BRAN MUFFINS WITH WALNUTS

READY IN ABOUT: 15 MIN

READY IN ABOUT: 20 MIN

SERVINGS: 12

Ingredients

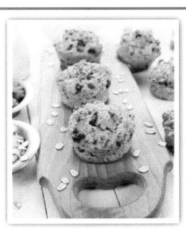

- 1 1/2 cups oat bran
- 1 cup whole wheat flour
- 1/2 cup chopped walnuts
- 1/3 cup honey or maple syrup
- 1/4 cup melted coconut oil or unsalted butter
- 1 cup unsweetened applesauce
- 2 eggs
- 1 tsp baking powder
- 1/2 tsp baking soda
- 1/2 tsp cinnamon
- 1/4 tsp salt

Directions

1. Preheat the oven. Use paper liners or food spray to grease a 12-cup muffin tin.
2. Mix oat bran, whole wheat flour, baking powder, baking soda, cinnamon & salt in a large basin. Melt coconut oil, honey, applesauce, and eggs in a separate bowl.
3. Mix the wet and dry components. Add the chopped walnuts and mix. Fill each muffin cup 2/3 full with batter.
4. A toothpick inserted into a muffin should come clean after 18–20 minutes.
5. After 5 minutes, move the muffins to a wire rack to cool fully.

PEANUT BUTTER AND BANANA OVERNIGHT OATS

READY IN ABOUT: 5 MIN

READY IN ABOUT: 0 MIN

SERVINGS: 2

Ingredients

- 1 cup rolled oats
- 1 cup unsweetened almond milk
- 1/2 cup Greek yogurt without added sugar
- 1 ripe banana, mashed
- 2 tbsp peanut butter
- 1 tbsp chia seeds
- 1 tbsp honey or maple syrup (optional)

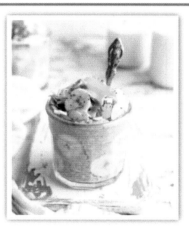

Directions

1. Mix the oats, milk, yogurt, banana, peanut butter, chia seeds, and sugar (if using) in a dish or container.
2. Freeze, covered, for at least 6 hours, preferably overnight.
3. Divide the oats evenly between two dishes and toss them before serving. Slice some bananas and sprinkle some peanut butter on top if you like.

PROTEIN-PACKED VEGGIE SCRAMBLE

READY IN ABOUT: 10 MIN

READY IN ABOUT: 10 MIN

SERVINGS: 1

Ingredients

- 2 eggs
- 1/4 cup cooked quinoa
- 1/2 cup chopped bell pepper
- 1/2 cup chopped tomato
- 1/4 cup diced onion
- 1/4 cup shredded cheese (optional)
- 1 tbsp olive oil
- Salt and pepper, to taste

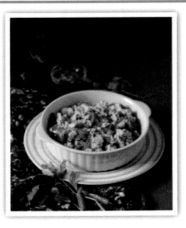

Directions

1. In a bowl, whisk the eggs and season with salt and pepper. In a non-stick skillet, warm the olive oil over moderate heat. Add the onions, bell pepper, and tomato, and cook for 5 minutes or until softened.
2. Stir in the cooked quinoa and cook for another 2 minutes. Pour the whisked eggs over the vegetables and quinoa, stirring to combine. Cook for 3-4 mins until the eggs are set.
3. Sprinkle cheese (if using) on top and cook for another 1-2 minutes to melt the cheese. Transfer the scramble to a plate and serve immediately.

BAKED BLUEBERRY OATMEAL

READY IN ABOUT: 10 MIN

READY IN ABOUT: 35 MIN

SERVINGS: 4

Ingredients

- 2 cups rolled oats
- 1 cup fresh or frozen blueberries
- 2 cups unsweetened almond milk
- 1/4 cup honey or maple syrup
- 1/4 cup unsweetened applesauce
- 1 tsp baking powder
- 1 tsp vanilla extract
- 1/2 tsp cinnamon
- Pinch of salt

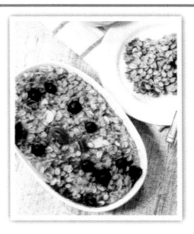

Directions

1. Set up the oven to 375°F (190°C). Grease an 8-inch square baking dish. Roll oats, baking powder, cinnamon, and salt in a large bowl.
2. Mix almond milk, honey, applesauce, and vanilla extract in a separate bowl.
3. Add and stir the wet ingredients to the dry ingredients until well combined. Combine the blueberries with the mixture.
4. Spatula-smooth the oatmeal mixture in the baking dish. Bake for 35-40 mins until oatmeal is set and rims are golden brown. Slice and serve after cooling.

QUINOA BREAKFAST BOWL WITH BERRIES

READY IN ABOUT: 5 MIN

READY IN ABOUT: 15 MIN

SERVINGS: 2

Ingredients

- 1/2 cup uncooked quinoa
- 1 cup water
- 1 cup mixed berries (fresh or frozen)
- 1/4 cup chopped nuts
- 1/4 cup unsweetened coconut flakes
- 1/4 cup Greek yogurt
- 2 tbsp honey or maple syrup (optional)

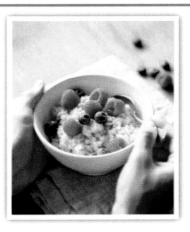

Directions

1. Drain the quinoa after giving it a good washing in cold water. Quinoa and water in a small saucepan. Take to a boil, then turn the heat low, cover, and simmer for 12-15 minutes until the quinoa is cooked and water is absorbed.
2. Set the pot aside for 5 minutes. Fluff the quinoa with a fork.
3. Divide the cooked quinoa between two bowls. Top each bowl with mixed berries, chopped nuts, coconut flakes, and a dollop of Greek yogurt.
4. Drizzle honey or maple syrup (if using) over the top of each bowl and serve.

AVOCADO AND EGG BREAKFAST BURRITO

READY IN ABOUT: 10 MIN

READY IN ABOUT: 10 MIN

SERVINGS: 2

Ingredients

- 2 large whole-grain tortillas
- 4 eggs
- 1 avocado, sliced
- 1/2 cup chopped tomato
- 1/4 cup diced onion
- 1/4 cup shredded cheese (optional)
- 1 tbsp olive oil
- Salt and pepper, to taste

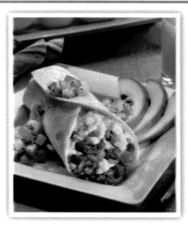

Directions

1. Whisk eggs with salt and pepper in a bowl. Heat olive oil on medium in a non-stick skillet. Cook onions for 3–4 minutes until tender.
2. Stir in the whisked eggs. Cook for 3–4 minutes or until the eggs are set.
3. If you're using cheese, sprinkle it on the eggs and cook for another minute or two to melt it.
4. Microwave or dry skillet the tortillas for 10-15 seconds on each side. Scramble eggs and divide them between tortillas. Add avocado slices and diced tomato.
5. Wrap the tortilla around the filling and roll it up to make a burrito. Slice in half and serve right away.

SPINACH AND FETA BREAKFAST WRAP

READY IN ABOUT: 10 MIN

READY IN ABOUT: 5 MIN

SERVINGS: 2

Ingredients

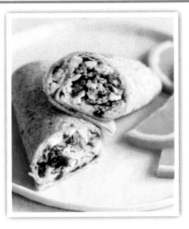

- 2 large whole-grain tortillas
- 4 eggs
- 2 cups fresh spinach
- 1/2 cup crumbled feta cheese
- 1/4 cup diced onion
- 1 tbsp olive oil
- Salt and pepper, to taste

Directions

1. Salt and pepper the eggs while you whisk them in a large mixing basin.
2. Heat olive oil on medium in a non-stick skillet. Cook onions for 3–4 minutes until tender.
3. Add the spinach to the pan and prepare for about two to three minutes or until it has softened.
4. Stir in the whisked eggs over the spinach and onions. Set eggs in 3–4 minutes. Mix in the broken pieces of feta cheese.
5. Microwave or dry skillet the tortillas for 10-15 seconds on each side.
6. Split the spinach-egg mixture between the tortillas. Roll the tortilla tightly over the filling. Cut in half and serve immediately.

PUMPKIN PIE SMOOTHIE

READY IN ABOUT: 5 MIN

READY IN ABOUT: 0 MIN

SERVINGS: 2

Ingredients

- 1 cup canned pumpkin puree (unsweetened)
- 1 cup unsweetened almond milk
- 1/2 cup Greek yogurt without added sugar
- 1 ripe banana
- 1 tsp pumpkin pie spice
- 1 tbsp honey or maple syrup (optional)
- 1 cup ice (optional)

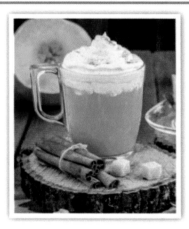

Directions

1. Combine the pumpkin puree, almond milk, Greek yogurt, banana, pumpkin pie spice, sweetener (if using), and ice (if using).
2. Blend until smooth and creamy.
3. Pour into two glasses and enjoy immediately.

CHOCOLATE CHERRY OVERNIGHT OATS

READY IN ABOUT: 5 MIN

READY IN ABOUT: 0 MIN

SERVINGS: 2

Ingredients

- 1 cup rolled oats
- 1 cup unsweetened almond milk
- 1/2 cup Greek yogurt
- 1/2 cup fresh or frozen cherries, pitted and chopped
- 2 tbsp unsweetened cocoa powder
- 1 tbsp chia seeds
- 1 tbsp honey or maple syrup (optional)

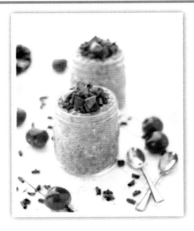

Directions

1. Mix the rolled oats, almond milk, Greek yogurt, cocoa powder, chia seeds, and (if you're using it) sugar in a bowl or jar.
2. Cover and put in the fridge for 6 hours or overnight. When you're ready to eat, stir the oats and split them between two bowls. Add chopped cherries on top, and enjoy!

TROPICAL GREEN SMOOTHIE

READY IN ABOUT: 5 MIN

READY IN ABOUT: 0 MIN

SERVINGS: 2

Ingredients

- 1 cup fresh spinach
- 1 cup unsweetened coconut milk
- 1 ripe banana
- 1 cup frozen mango chunks
- 1 cup frozen pineapple chunks
- 1 tbsp chia seeds

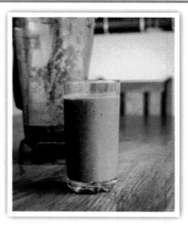

Directions

1. Combine the spinach, coconut milk, banana, mango, pineapple, and chia seeds in a blender.
2. Blend until smooth and creamy.
3. Pour into two glasses and enjoy immediately.

BAKED AVOCADO EGG BOATS

READY IN ABOUT: 5 MIN

READY IN ABOUT: 15-18 MIN

SERVINGS: 2

Ingredients

- 1 ripe avocado, halved and pitted
- 2 eggs
- Salt and pepper, to taste
- Optional toppings: crumbled feta cheese, chopped chives, hot sauce

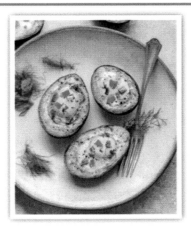

Directions

1. Set up the oven to 425°F (220°C). To make a larger egg well, scoop avocado flesh from either half. Place avocado halves on a baking sheet or small oven-safe dish.
2. Crack eggs into avocado halves. Salt and pepper.
3. Bake for 15-18 minutes until the egg whites are set, and the yolks are done to your liking.
4. Add your toppings after baking. Serve immediately.

VEGGIE BREAKFAST SKILLET

READY IN ABOUT: 10 MIN

READY IN ABOUT: 20 MIN

SERVINGS: 2

Ingredients

- 1 medium sweet potato, peeled and diced
- 1/2 cup chopped bell pepper
- 1/2 cup chopped tomato
- 1/4 cup diced onion
- 2 cups fresh spinach
- 4 eggs
- 2 tbsp olive oil
- Salt and pepper, to taste

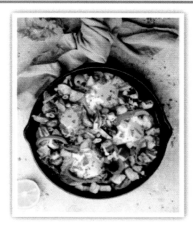

Directions

1. In a large non-stick pan, warm the olive oil over a medium-high flame. Cook the diced sweet potato for 10-12 minutes, stirring regularly, until soft and slightly browned.
2. Cook the onions and bell pepper in the skillet for 3-4 minutes until softened. Add chopped tomato and simmer for 2 more minutes.
3. Wilt the spinach in the skillet for 2-3 minutes. Put an egg in each of the four veggie mixture wells. Salt and pepper.
4. Cover the skillet for 5-7 minutes to set the egg whites and cook the yolks to your liking.
5. Serve immediately.

GRILLED SALMON SALAD WITH AVOCADO

READY IN ABOUT: 10 MIN

READY IN ABOUT: 10 MIN

SERVINGS: 2

Ingredients

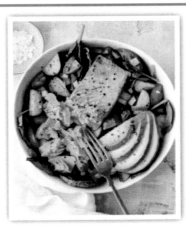

- 2 salmon fillets (4-6 oz each)
- 4 cups mixed greens
- 1 avocado, sliced
- 1/2 cup cherry tomatoes, halved
- 1/4 cup red onion, thinly sliced
- 1/4 cup chopped walnuts
- Olive oil
- Salt and pepper, to taste

For the dressing

- 3 tbsp olive oil
- 2 tbsp lemon juice
- 1 tsp Dijon mustard
- 1 tsp honey or maple syrup (optional)
- Salt and pepper, to taste

Directions

1. Heat a grill to medium-high. Apply olive oil to the salmon fillets in a rubbing motion and season with salt & pepper to taste.
2. Grill salmon for 4-5 minutes per side until it flakes easily. Mixed greens, avocado, cherry tomatoes, red onion, and walnuts in a large bowl.
3. Mix the dressing ingredients in a bowl. Season to taste. After adding the sauce, stir the salad to mix it.
4. Serve the salad with grilled salmon on two plates.

CHICKPEA AND QUINOA STUFFED BELL PEPPERS

READY IN ABOUT: 15 MIN

READY IN ABOUT: 30 MIN

SERVINGS: 4

Ingredients

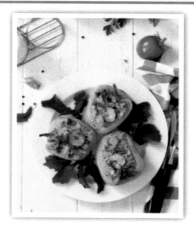

- 4 bell peppers, halved lengthwise and seeds removed
- 1 cup cooked quinoa
- 1 cup canned chickpeas, drained and rinsed
- 1 cup cherry tomatoes, halved
- 1/2 cup diced cucumber
- 1/4 cup crumbled feta cheese (optional)
- 1/4 cup chopped parsley
- 2 tbsp olive oil
- 1 tbsp lemon juice
- Salt and pepper, to taste

Directions

1. Set the oven's temperature to 375°F (190°C). Parchment a baking sheet.
2. Olive oil and the bell pepper halves on the baking sheet. Salt and pepper are used as seasonings.
3. Mix the cooked quinoa, chickpeas, cherry tomatoes, cucumber, feta, parsley, olive oil, and lemon juice in a large bowl. Toss salt and pepper.
4. Spoon the quinoa blending into the bell pepper halves and fill them with gentle pressure.
5. Prepare for 25–30 mins until the peppers are cooked, and the quinoa is warm. Serve warm or at room temperature.

LENTIL SOUP WITH TURMERIC AND GINGER

READY IN ABOUT: 10 MIN

READY IN ABOUT: 40 MIN

SERVINGS: 4

Ingredients

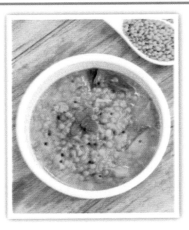

- 1 cup brown lentils, rinsed and drained
- 6 cups vegetable broth
- 1 onion, diced
- 2 carrots, chopped
- 2 celery stalks, chopped
- 2 cloves garlic, minced
- 1 tsp ground turmeric
- 1 tsp grated fresh ginger
- 1 tsp ground cumin
- 1/2 tsp ground coriander
- Salt and pepper, to taste
- 2 tbsp olive oil

Directions

1. Medium-heat olive oil in a big pot. Cook onion, carrots, and celery for 5-7 minutes until softened.
2. Cook the garlic, turmeric, ginger, cumin, and coriander for another 1-2 minutes until fragrant.
3. Mix lentils with vegetable broth. Take to a boil, then decrease the heat to low and saute until lentils are cooked, 30–40 minutes. Salt and pepper the soup to taste. Serve with Greek yogurt or cilantro.

KALE AND SWEET POTATO SALAD

READY IN ABOUT: 10 MIN

READY IN ABOUT: 25 MIN

SERVINGS: 4

Ingredients

- 1 large sweet potato, peeled and diced
- 1 bunch, kale, stems removed and chopped
- 1/2 cup cooked quinoa
- 1/4 cup dried cranberries
- 1/4 cup chopped walnuts
- 3 tbsp olive oil, divided
- Salt and pepper, to taste
- For the dressing:
- 2 tbsp olive oil
- 1 tbsp apple cider vinegar
- 1 tsp Dijon mustard
- 1 tsp honey or maple syrup (optional)
- Salt and pepper, to taste

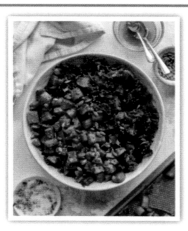

Directions

1. Turn the oven's heat to 400°F (200°C). Parchment a baking sheet.
2. Pour 1 tablespoon olive oil over the chopped sweet potato on the baking sheet. Add salt and pepper to taste. Roast for 20–25 mins or until soft and lightly browned.
3. Massage chopped kale with 2 tablespoons olive oil in a large basin until tender. Whisk to mix all of the ingredients for the dressing in a bowl. Season to taste.
4. Mix the kale with the cooked rice, roasted sweet potato, dried cranberries, and walnuts. Pour the dressing over the salad and swirl to combine it.
5. Spread the salad out evenly across four dishes and serve.

SPICED CAULIFLOWER RICE WITH TOFU

READY IN ABOUT: 10 MIN

READY IN ABOUT: 20 MIN

SERVINGS: 4

Ingredients

- 1 head of cauliflower, chopped into florets
- 1 block of firm tofu, drained and cubed
- 2 cups chopped bell pepper
- 1 cup frozen peas, thawed
- 1/4 cup chopped green onions
- 2 cloves garlic, minced
- 1 tsp ground cumin
- 1 tsp ground turmeric
- 1/2 tsp ground ginger
- Salt and pepper, to taste
- 3 tbsp olive oil, divided

Directions

1. Pulse cauliflower florets in a blender until rice-like. Put aside. Over moderate heat, warm 2 tablespoons of oil in a big nonstick skillet. Cook the tofu for 8-10 minutes, stirring regularly, until browned on all sides. Set aside the tofu.
2. Warm the last tbsp of olive oil in the skillet. Cook the bell pepper for 5 minutes until tender.
3. Add garlic, cumin, turmeric, and ginger and simmer for 1 minute until aromatic.
4. Cook the cauliflower rice and peas in the skillet for 5-7 minutes, stirring regularly, until cooked.
5. Mix in the tofu. Salt & pepper to taste. Serve the cauliflower rice atop with green onions.

MEDITERRANEAN ORZO SALAD

READY IN ABOUT: 15 MIN

READY IN ABOUT: 10 MIN

SERVINGS: 4

Ingredients

- 1 cup uncooked orzo pasta
- 1 cup cherry tomatoes, halved
- 1 cup chopped cucumber
- 1/2 cup of Kalamata olive, pitted and cut in half
- 1/2 cup crumbled feta cheese (optional)
- 1/4 cup chopped fresh basil
- 1/4 cup chopped fresh parsley
- 1/4 cup olive oil
- 2 tbsp lemon juice
- Salt and pepper, to taste

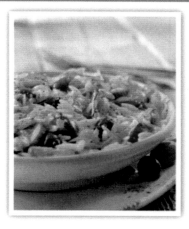

Directions

1. Cook the orzo as per the package instructions. Drain and rinse under chilled water to cool.
2. Combine the cooked orzo, cherry tomatoes, cucumber, olives, feta (if using), basil, and parsley in a large bowl.
3. Mix olive oil and then add lime juice in a small bowl. Season with salt & pepper to taste.
4. Combine the salad and dressing together with a toss. Serve right away or chill.

ZUCCHINI NOODLES WITH PESTO

READY IN ABOUT: 10 MIN

READY IN ABOUT: 5 MIN

SERVINGS: 2

Ingredients

- 2 medium zucchini
- 1/2 cup prepared basil pesto
- 1/2 cup cherry tomatoes, halved
- 1/4 cup grated Parmesan cheese (optional)
- Salt and pepper, to taste

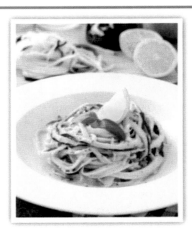

Directions

1. Spiralize or julienne zucchini to make noodles. Set aside.
2. Heat pesto in a large skillet on medium-low. Cook zucchini noodles for 2-3 minutes until tender.
3. Add the cherry tomatoes and heat for 1-2 minutes. Season with salt and pepper to taste. If desired, serve topped with grated Parmesan cheese.

BUTTERNUT SQUASH AND BLACK BEAN TACOS

READY IN ABOUT: 15 MIN

READY IN ABOUT: 30 MIN

SERVINGS: 4

Ingredients

- 2 cups cubed butternut squash
- 1 cup canned black beans, drained and washed
- 1/2 cup diced red onion
- 1/4 cup chopped fresh cilantro
- 1 tsp ground cumin
- 1 tsp smoked paprika
- Salt and pepper, to taste
- 2 tbsp olive oil
- 8 small corn or whole wheat tortillas
- Optional toppings: avocado, lime wedges, Greek yogurt

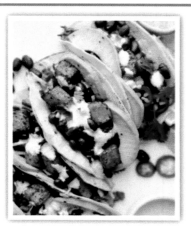

Directions

1. Set the oven's temperature to 400°F (200°C). Put parchment paper on a baking sheet. Mix the butternut squash, black beans, red onion, cumin, smoked paprika, salt & pepper in a big bowl. Drizzle olive oil on the vegetables and toss to coat.
2. Spread the blending on the baking sheet and bake for 25–30 mins until the squash gets soft and lightly browned.
3. To heat the tortillas, follow the instructions on the package.
4. Fill each tortilla with the roasted squash and black bean mixture, and top with chopped cilantro and any additional desired toppings. Serve immediately.
5. Please let me know which recipes you'd like to receive next, and I'll be happy to provide them.

THAI COCONUT CURRY WITH VEGETABLES

READY IN ABOUT: 15 MIN

READY IN ABOUT: 25 MIN

SERVINGS: 4

Ingredients

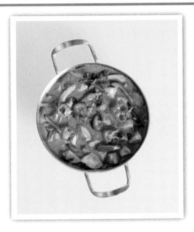

- 1 can (14 oz) full-fat coconut milk (without added sugar)
- 1 cup vegetable broth
- 2 cups chopped mixed vegetables (e.g., bell peppers, carrots, zucchini)
- 1 cup chopped kale or spinach
- 1/2 cup diced onion
- 2 cloves garlic, minced
- 1 tbsp Thai red curry paste
- 1 tbsp grated fresh ginger
- 1 tbsp soy sauce or tamari
- 1 tsp maple syrup (optional)
- 2 tbsp olive oil
- Salt and pepper, to taste
- Cooked rice for serving
- Fresh cilantro for garnish

Directions

1. In a big nonstick skillet on medium heat, warm the oil. Cook the onion for 3-4 mins until it gets softened. Add garlic, curry paste, and ginger and simmer for 1-2 minutes until aromatic.
2. Cook mixed vegetables for 5 minutes until tender. Mix the coconut milk, vegetable broth, soy sauce, and brown sugar. Take to a simmer, then decrease the heat to low and cook until vegetables get soft, 10-15 minutes.
3. Add chopped kale or spinach and simmer for 2-3 minutes until wilted. Salt & pepper to taste. Serve the curry over cooked rice, garnished with fresh cilantro.

SPINACH AND FETA STUFFED CHICKEN BREAST

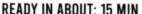

READY IN ABOUT: 15 MIN

READY IN ABOUT: 25 MIN

SERVINGS: 4

Ingredients

- 4 boneless, skinless chicken breasts
- 1 cup chopped fresh spinach
- 1/2 cup crumbled feta cheese (optional)
- 1/4 cup sun-dried tomatoes, chopped
- 2 cloves garlic, minced
- Salt and pepper, to taste
- 2 tbsp olive oil

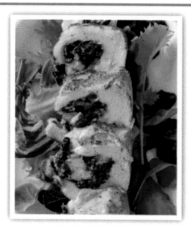

Directions

1. Turn the oven's heat to 375°F (190°C). Parchment a baking sheet. Spinach, feta, sun-dried tomatoes, and garlic in a small bowl.
2. Carefully cut a horizontal slit in each chicken breast. Fill each pocket with the spinach mixture, then use a toothpick to close the hole.
3. Add salt & pepper to the chicken breasts. Heat olive oil on a medium-sized in a large oven-safe skillet. Cook chicken breasts for 4-5 minutes per side till golden brown.
4. Prepare the skillet in the preheated oven for 15-20 minutes until the chicken is done and 165°F (74°C). Rest the chicken before serving.

MEDITERRANEAN QUINOA SALAD

READY IN ABOUT: 15 MIN

READY IN ABOUT: 15 MIN

SERVINGS: 4

Ingredients

- 1 cup uncooked quinoa
- 2 cups cherry tomatoes, halved
- 1 cup chopped cucumber
- 1/2 cup olives, pitted and cut in half
- 1/2 cup crumbled feta cheese (optional)
- 1/4 cup chopped fresh parsley
- 1/4 cup chopped fresh mint
- 1/4 cup olive oil
- 2 tbsp lemon juice
- Salt and pepper, to taste

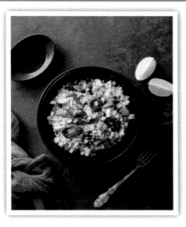

Directions

1. Cook quinoa as per package directions. Drain and chill under cold water.
2. Mix cooked quinoa, cherry tomatoes, cucumber, olives, feta, parsley, and mint in a large bowl.
3. In a bowl, combine oil and lemon juice. Season with salt and pepper to taste. Dress the salad and toss. Serve right away or chill.

CURRIED LENTIL AND RICE BOWL

READY IN ABOUT: 10 MIN

READY IN ABOUT: 40 MIN

SERVINGS: 4

Ingredients

- 1 cup uncooked brown rice
- 1 cup green dried lentils, washed and drained
- 1 cup diced carrots
- 1 cup diced bell pepper
- 1/2 cup chopped onion
- 1/4 cup raisins or currants
- 1/4 cup chopped fresh cilantro
- 2 cloves garlic, minced
- 1 tbsp curry powder
- 1 tsp ground cumin
- Salt and pepper, to taste
- 3 cups vegetable broth
- 2 tbsp olive oil

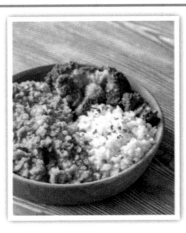

Directions

1. Warm olive oil in a big pot on medium-high flame. Cook the onion for 3-4 mins until it gets softened.
2. Add garlic, curry powder, and cumin and simmer for 1-2 minutes until fragrant. Stir in the brown rice and lentils. Boil the veggie broth.
3. Cover and cook on low for 30–35 mins til the rice and lentils are soft, and the liquid is absorbed.
4. Add the carrots, bell pepper, and raisins and simmer for 5 minutes until soft.
5. Season with salt and pepper to taste. Serve the lentil and rice mixture topped with chopped cilantro.

BROCCOLI SLAW WITH TAHINI DRESSING

READY IN ABOUT: 15 MIN

READY IN ABOUT: 0 MIN

SERVINGS: 4

Ingredients

- 4 cups broccoli slaw mix
- 1 cup shredded red cabbage
- 1/2 cup chopped green onions
- 1/4 cup chopped fresh cilantro
- 1/4 cup sesame seeds

For the dressing

- 1/4 cup tahini
- 2 tbsp lemon juice
- 1 tbsp honey or maple syrup
- 1 tbsp soy sauce or tamari
- 1 tbsp rice vinegar
- 1 tbsp olive oil
- 1 clove garlic, minced
- Salt and pepper, to taste

Directions

1. Mix broccoli slaw, red cabbage, green onions, cilantro, and sesame seeds in a large bowl.
2. Mix the dressing in a small bowl. Change the seasonings to your liking. Toss the dressing over the slaw. Serve it right away.

GREEK SALAD WITH GRILLED CHICKEN

READY IN ABOUT: 20 MIN

READY IN ABOUT: 10 MIN

SERVINGS: 4

Ingredients

- 4 boneless, skinless chicken breasts
- 1 head romaine lettuce, chopped
- 1 cup cherry tomatoes, halved
- 1 cup chopped cucumber
- 1/2 cup of olives, pitted and halved
- 1/2 cup crumbled feta cheese (optional)
- 1/4 cup chopped red onion
- 1/4 cup olive oil
- 2 tbsp lemon juice
- 1 tbsp dried oregano
- Salt and pepper, to taste

Directions

1. Preheat a grill or grill pan over medium heat. The chicken breasts are seasoned with salt, pepper, and oregano.
2. Grill the chicken for 5-6 mins per side until cooked through and 165°F (74°C). Slice after resting. Mix lettuce, cherry tomatoes, cucumber, olives, feta, and red onion
3. in a large bowl.
4. Olive oil and lime juice are combined in a large basin. Season to flavor with salt and pepper.
5. Drizzle the dressing over the salad and incorporate it with a toss. Serve with grilled chicken.

ROASTED BEET AND GOAT CHEESE SALAD

READY IN ABOUT: 15 MIN

READY IN ABOUT: 60 MIN

SERVINGS: 4

Ingredients

- 4 medium beets, scrubbed and trimmed
- 1/2 cup crumbled goat cheese (optional)
- 1/4 cup chopped walnuts
- 1/4 cup chopped fresh mint
- 1/4 cup olive oil
- 2 tbsp balsamic vinegar
- Salt and pepper, to taste

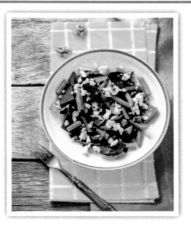

Directions

1. Set the heat of your oven to 400°F (200°C). Individually wrap each beet in aluminum foil and place it on a baking sheet. Roast until fork-tender, 1 hour. Let the beets cool before peeling and cutting them into wedges.
2. Mix beet wedges, goat cheese, walnuts, and mint in a large bowl.
3. In a mixing bowl, incorporate together olive oil and balsamic vinegar. Add a little salt & pepper to taste. Put the sauce over the salad and stir it up. Serve right away.

WARM GRAIN SALAD WITH ROASTED VEGETABLES

READY IN ABOUT: 20 MIN

READY IN ABOUT: 25 MIN

SERVINGS: 4

Ingredients

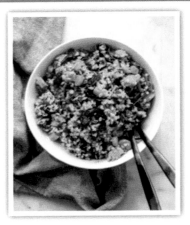

- 1 cup uncooked farro, barley, or other whole grain
- 2 cups chopped vegetables (e.g., zucchini, bell pepper, onion, cherry tomatoes)
- 1/4 cup chopped fresh parsley
- 1/4 cup chopped fresh basil
- 1/4 cup olive oil
- 2 tbsp lemon juice
- Salt and pepper, to taste

Directions

1. Cook grain according to package directions. Drain and put away. Start the oven at 425°F (220°C). Cover a baking sheet with parchment paper.
2. Mix vegetables with 1 tablespoon olive oil and salt and pepper. Roast the veggies on a baking sheet for 20–25 mins, or until they are soft and just beginning to brown.
3. A large bowl of cooked grain, roasted vegetables, parsley, and basil. Mix the rest of the olive oil and lime juice in a small bowl. Salt & pepper to taste.
4. Pour the dressing over the grains and vegetables and mix. The salad can be served hot or at room temperature.

COLD SOBA NOODLE SALAD

READY IN ABOUT: 20 MIN

READY IN ABOUT: 5 MIN

SERVINGS: 4

Ingredients

- 8 oz soba noodles
- 1 cup julienned carrots
- 1 cup julienned bell pepper
- 1 cup thinly sliced cucumber
- 1/2 cup chopped green onions
- 1/4 cup chopped fresh cilantro
- 1/4 cup chopped fresh basil
- 1/4 cup soy sauce or tamari
- 2 tbsp rice vinegar
- 2 tbsp sesame oil
- 1 tbsp honey or maple syrup
- 1 tbsp grated fresh ginger
- 1 clove garlic, minced

Directions

1. To cook the soba noodles, follow the instructions on the package. Drain and chill under cold water.
2. Mix cooked noodles, carrots, bell pepper, cucumber, green onions, cilantro, and basil in a large bowl.
3. Mix soy sauce, rice vinegar, sesame oil, honey, ginger, and garlic in a small bowl.
4. Toss the dressing over the noodles. Serve salad chilled or at room temperature.

ASIAN CHICKEN LETTUCE WRAPS

READY IN ABOUT: 15 MIN

READY IN ABOUT: 10 MIN

SERVINGS: 4

Ingredients

- 1 lb ground chicken or turkey
- 1/2 cup diced onion
- 1/2 cup diced bell pepper
- 1/2 cup grated carrots
- 2 cloves garlic, minced
- 1/4 cup hoisin sauce
- 2 tbsp soy sauce or tamari
- 1 tbsp rice vinegar
- 1 tbsp grated fresh ginger
- 1 tbsp sesame oil
- Salt and pepper, to taste
- 1 head butter lettuce, leaves separated

Directions

1. Medium-heat sesame oil in a big skillet. Cook the onion for 3-4 mins until it gets softened.
2. Break up and fry the ground chicken or turkey in the skillet. Add garlic, bell pepper, and carrots and simmer for 2-3 minutes.
3. Mix hoisin, soy, rice vinegar, and ginger in a small bowl. The chicken is ready after 2 minutes in the microwave with the sauce.
4. Serve the chicken mixture in the lettuce leaves, wrapping them up like tacos. Enjoy!

STUFFED AVOCADO WITH TUNA

READY IN ABOUT: 15 MIN

READY IN ABOUT: 0 MIN

SERVINGS: 2

Ingredients

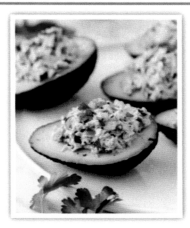

- 1 large avocado, halved and pitted
- 1 can (5 oz) tuna, drained and flaked
- 1/4 cup diced cucumber
- 1/4 cup diced red bell pepper
- 1/4 cup chopped fresh cilantro
- 1/4 cup Greek yogurt (without added sugar)or mayonnaise
- 1 tbsp lemon juice
- Salt and pepper, to taste

Directions

1. Combine the tuna, cucumber, bell pepper, cilantro, yogurt or mayonnaise, and lemon juice in a medium bowl. Season with salt and pepper to taste.
2. Spoon the tuna mixture onto the avocado halves, filling the cavity where the pit was removed. Serve immediately.

RAINBOW VEGGIE COLLARD WRAPS

READY IN ABOUT: 20 MIN

READY IN ABOUT: 0 MIN

SERVINGS: 4

Ingredients

- 8 large collard green leaves, stems removed
- 1 cup hummus
- 1 cup grated carrots
- 1 cup thinly sliced bell pepper
- 1 cup thinly sliced cucumber
- 1 cup thinly sliced red cabbage
- 1 cup alfalfa sprouts or microgreens
- Salt and pepper, to taste

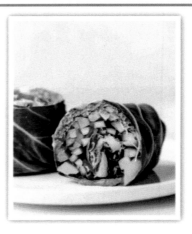

Directions

1. Place the collard green leaves in a basin of ice water to stop cooking after boiling them for 30 seconds. Use a clean towel to dry the leaves.
2. Lay a collard green leaf flat on a cutting board or plate, and spread about 2 tablespoons of hummus onto the center of the leaf.
3. Layer the hummus over the carrots, bell pepper, cucumber, red cabbage, and sprouts or microgreens. Season with salt and pepper to taste.
4. Gently fold the sides of the collard leaf over the filling, then roll the leaf up from the bottom to create a wrap. Repeat with the remaining collard leaves and filling ingredients.
5. Serve the wraps whole or slice them in half to reveal the colorful layers. Enjoy!

BLACK BEAN AND CORN SALAD

READY IN ABOUT: 15 MIN

READY IN ABOUT: 0 MIN

SERVINGS: 4

Ingredients

- 1 pack (15 oz) of black beans, drained and washed
- 1 cup cooked corn kernels (fresh)
- 1 cup diced bell pepper
- 1/2 cup diced red onion
- 1/2 cup chopped fresh cilantro
- 1/4 cup olive oil
- 2 tbsp lime juice
- 1 tsp ground cumin
- Salt and pepper, to taste

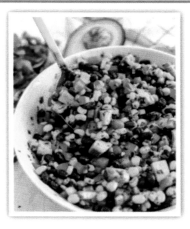

Directions

1. Combine the black beans, corn, bell pepper, red onion, and cilantro in a large bowl.
2. Mix olive oil, lime juice, and cumin in a small mixing bowl; season with pepper and salt to taste.
3. Pour the dressing over the bean-corn mixture and mix. Serve the salad immediately or chill.

ROASTED VEGETABLE QUINOA BOWLS

READY IN ABOUT: 20 MIN

READY IN ABOUT: 30 MIN

SERVINGS: 4

Ingredients

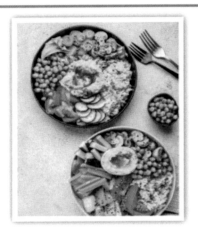

- 1 cup uncooked quinoa
- 2 cups chopped vegetables (e.g., zucchini, bell pepper, cherry tomatoes, red onion)
- 1 pack (15 oz) chickpeas, drained and rinsed
- 1/4 cup olive oil
- 2 tbsp balsamic vinegar
- 1 tbsp fresh lemon juice
- 1 tsp dried oregano
- Salt and pepper, to taste
- Optional toppings: crumbled feta cheese, chopped fresh parsley, sliced avocado

Directions

1. Set the oven's temperature to 425°F (220°C) and turn it on. Put parchment paper on a baking sheet.
2. Cook quinoa per package directions. Drain and put away.
3. Toss vegetables and chickpeas with 1 tablespoon of olive oil and salt and pepper. Roast the mixture on the prepared baking sheet for 25–30 minutes until soft and gently browned.
4. Mix the remaining olive oil, balsamic vinegar, lemon juice, and oregano in a separate dish. Salt & pepper to taste.
5. Divide the cooked quinoa among four bowls, and top with the roasted vegetables and chickpeas. Drizzle with the dressing and garnish with your choice of optional toppings.

TURKEY AND VEGGIE STUFFED BELL PEPPERS

READY IN ABOUT: 1 MIN

READY IN ABOUT: 30 MIN

SERVINGS: 4

Ingredients

- 4 large bell peppers, tops removed and seeds discarded
- 1 lb ground turkey
- 1 cup cooked brown rice
- 1 cup chopped vegetables (e.g., zucchini, onion, mushrooms)
- 1 can (15 oz) diced tomatoes, drained
- 1/4 cup chopped fresh basil
- 1/4 cup grated Parmesan cheese (optional)
- 1 tbsp olive oil
- Salt and pepper, to taste

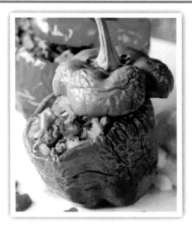

Directions

1. Turn your oven's heat to 375°F (190°C). Grease a bell pepper-sized baking dish. In a large nonstick pot, warm the olive oil over moderate heat. Add the ground turkey and brown it, tearing it up with a spoon.
2. Cook veggies for 3–4 minutes. Stir cooked rice, diced tomatoes, and basil into the skillet. Salt & pepper to taste.
3. Fill bell peppers with turkey-rice mixture. Put the stuffed peppers in the dish set up for baking.
4. Bake for 25–30 mins until peppers are tender and filling is cooked.
5. If desired, sprinkle the peppers with Parmesan cheese during the last 5 minutes of baking. Serve the stuffed peppers warm.

SPICY LENTIL AND SWEET POTATO STEW

READY IN ABOUT: 15 MIN

READY IN ABOUT: 45 MIN

SERVINGS: 4

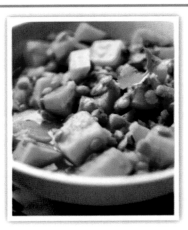

Ingredients

- 1 tbsp olive oil
- 1 onion, chopped
- 2 cloves garlic, minced
- 1 tbsp grated fresh ginger
- 1 tsp ground cumin
- 1 tsp ground coriander
- 1 tsp ground turmeric
- 1/4 tsp cayenne pepper to taste
- 1 1/2 cups brown lentils, rinsed and drained
- 4 cups vegetable broth
- 2 medium sweet potatoes, peeled and diced
- 1 can (14 oz) diced tomatoes
- 1/4 cup chopped fresh cilantro
- Salt and pepper, to taste
- Optional toppings: Greek yogurt or sour cream, additional cilantro, sliced

Directions

1. Warm the olive oil over a moderate-high flame in a large pot or Dutch oven. Cook the onion for 3-4 mins until it gets softened.
2. Add garlic, ginger, cumin, coriander, turmeric, and cayenne. Cook until fragrant.
3. Add lentils, vegetable broth, sweet potatoes, and diced tomatoes to the pot. After boiling, decrease the heat and simmer for 30–40 minutes until the lentils and sweet potatoes are cooked.
4. Stir in the chopped cilantro and season the stew with salt and pepper to taste.
5. Serve the stew hot, garnished with your choice of optional toppings.

CHICKPEA AND SPINACH CURRY

READY IN ABOUT: 10 MIN

READY IN ABOUT: 25 MIN

SERVINGS: 4

Ingredients

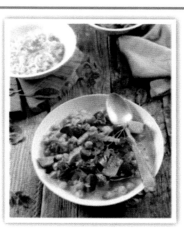

- 1 tbsp coconut oil
- 1 onion, chopped
- 2 cloves garlic, minced
- 1 tbsp grated fresh ginger
- 1 tbsp curry powder
- 1 tsp ground turmeric
- 1/2 tsp ground cumin
- 1 can (15 oz.) chickpeas, drained and washed
- 1 can (14 oz) diced tomatoes
- 1 can (14 oz) coconut milk
- 4 cups fresh spinach
- Salt and pepper, to taste
- Optional toppings: chopped fresh cilantro, sliced almonds, raisins

Directions

1. Warm the coconut oil over moderate heat in a big skillet. Cook the onion for 3-4 mins until it gets softened.
2. Mix garlic, ginger, curry powder, turmeric, and cumin. Cook for another min or two or until the smell is nice.
3. Add chickpeas, diced tomatoes, and coconut milk to a skillet. After boiling, turn down the heat and prepare for 15-20 mins to blend the flavors.
4. Add spinach and simmer for 3–4 minutes until wilted. Salt and pepper the curry to taste.
5. Serve the curry hot, garnished with your choice of optional toppings.

GINGER-SESAME BAKED SALMON

READY IN ABOUT: 10 MIN

READY IN ABOUT: 15 MIN

SERVINGS: 4

Ingredients

- 4 (6 oz) salmon fillets
- 1/4 cup low-sodium soy sauce
- 1/4 cup honey or maple syrup
- 1 tbsp grated fresh ginger
- 1 tbsp sesame oil
- 1 tbsp rice vinegar
- 2 cloves garlic, minced
- 1 tbsp sesame seeds
- 2 green onions, thinly sliced
- Salt and pepper, to taste

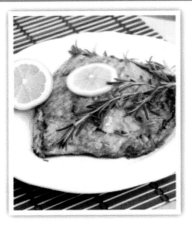

Directions

1. Prepare a hot oven by setting the temperature to 400°F (200 degrees C). Prepare a parchment paper-lined baking sheet.
2. Mix soy sauce, honey, ginger, sesame oil, rice vinegar, and garlic in a small bowl.
3. Salt and pepper the salmon fillets on the baking sheet. Spread the sauce on each salmon fillet.
4. Make sure the salmon is cooked through by baking it for 12-15 minutes.
5. Sprinkle the cooked salmon with sesame seeds and green onions. Serve the salmon hot, drizzled with any remaining sauce from the baking sheet.

LEMON HERB GRILLED SHRIMP

READY IN ABOUT: 15 MIN

READY IN ABOUT: 6-8 MIN

SERVINGS: 4

Ingredients

- 1 lb large shrimp, peeled and deveined
- 1/4 cup olive oil
- 3 cloves garlic, minced
- Zest and juice of 1 lemon
- 2 tbsp chopped fresh parsley
- 1 tbsp chopped fresh basil
- 1 tsp dried oregano
- Salt and pepper, to taste

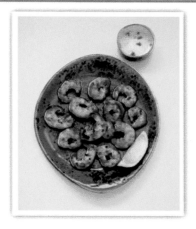

Directions

1. Whisk together the olive oil, garlic, lemon zest, lemon juice, parsley, basil, oregano, salt & pepper in a large bowl.
2. Toss the shrimp in the bowl to coat them. Allow the shrimp to stay marinated in the refrigerator for 15-30 mins.
3. Preheat a grill or grill pan to medium-high heat. Thread the shrimp onto skewers, if desired.
4. Grill the shrimp for 3-4 mins per side or until cooked through and opaque. If desired, serve the grilled shrimp hot, garnished with additional chopped herbs.

AKED ZUCCHINI BOATS WITH QUINOA AND TOMATOES

READY IN ABOUT: 15 MIN

READY IN ABOUT: 35 MIN

SERVINGS: 4

Ingredients

- 4 medium zucchini
- 1 cup cooked quinoa
- 1 cup cherry tomatoes, halved
- 1/2 cup crumbled feta cheese
- 1/4 cup chopped fresh basil
- 2 cloves garlic, minced
- 1 tbsp olive oil
- Salt and pepper, to taste

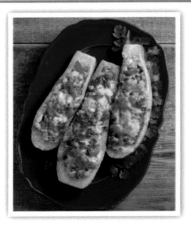

Directions

1. Set up the oven to 400°F (200°C). Line a sheet pan with parchment paper. Half the zucchini lengthwise and use a spoon to dig out the seeds and meat, leaving a 1/4-inch shell. Put the halves of the zucchini on the baking sheet.
2. Combine the cooked quinoa, cherry tomatoes, feta cheese, basil, garlic, olive oil, salt, and pepper in a large bowl.
3. Spoon the quinoa mixture into the zucchini boats, pressing slightly to fill the cavity. Bake the zucchini boats for 30-35 minutes until the zucchini is tender, and the quinoa mixture is golden brown.
4. If desired, serve the zucchini boats hot, garnished with additional chopped basil.

CAULIFLOWER STEAKS WITH CHIMICHURRI SAUCE

READY IN ABOUT: 15 MIN

READY IN ABOUT: 20 MIN

SERVINGS: 4

Ingredients

- 1 large head of cauliflower
- 1/4 cup olive oil, divided
- Salt and pepper, to taste
- 1 cup fresh parsley leaves
- 1/2 cup fresh cilantro leaves
- 2 cloves garlic, minced
- 1/4 cup red wine vinegar
- 1/2 tsp crushed red pepper flakes

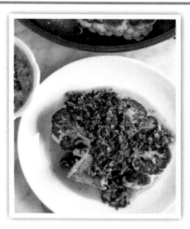

Directions

1. Set up the temperature of the oven to 425°F (220°C). Line a baking tray with parchment paper. Trim the cauliflower stem and outer leaves, leaving the core. Cut cauliflower into 1-inch steaks.
2. Season cauliflower steaks with salt and olive oil. Place the steaks on the prepared baking tray. Bake the cauliflower steaks for 20-25 minutes or until tender and golden brown, flipping halfway through cooking.
3. While the cauliflower is baking, prepare the chimichurri sauce. Combine the parsley, cilantro, garlic, red wine vinegar, crushed red pepper flakes, and olive oil in a food processor. Process until smooth, and season with salt and pepper, to taste.
4. Serve the cauliflower steaks hot, drizzled with the chimichurri sauce.

COD WITH TOMATO AND OLIVE TAPENADE

READY IN ABOUT: 15 MIN

READY IN ABOUT: 15 MIN

SERVINGS: 4

Ingredients

- 4 cod fillets, 6 ounces each
- Salt and pepper, to taste
- 1 tbsp olive oil
- 2 cups cherry tomatoes, halved
- 1/2 cup pitted Kalamata olives, chopped
- 1/4 cup chopped fresh parsley
- 1 clove garlic, minced
- Zest and juice of 1 lemon

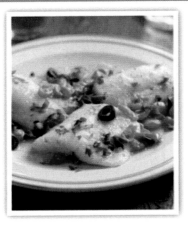

Directions

1. Set the oven's temperature to 400°F (200°C). Line a sheet pan with parchment paper. Place the salted and peppered cod fillets on the baking sheet.
2. In a medium bowl, combine olive oil, cherry tomatoes, Kalamata olives, parsley, garlic, lemon zest, and lime juice.
3. Press the tomato-olive mixture onto the fish fillets. Bake the cod until it flakes readily with a fork , 12 to 15 minutes.
4. Serve the cod hot, topped with any remaining tomato and olive mixture from the baking sheet.

LENTIL AND VEGETABLE STUFFED PEPPERS

READY IN ABOUT: 20 MIN

READY IN ABOUT: 45 MIN

SERVINGS: 4

Ingredients

- 4 large bell peppers, any color
- 2 cups cooked green or brown lentils
- 1 cup chopped fresh spinach
- 1/2 cup diced red onion
- 1/2 cup crumbled feta cheese
- 1/4 cup chopped fresh basil
- 2 cloves garlic, minced
- 1 tbsp olive oil
- Salt and pepper, to taste

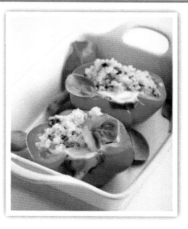

Directions

1. Set the oven's temperature to 375°F (190°C). Line a baking dish with parchment paper.
2. Remove the seeds and skins from the bell peppers and cut off the tops. Place the peppers upright in the prepared baking dish.
3. Combine the cooked lentils, spinach, red onion, feta cheese, basil, garlic, olive oil, salt, and pepper in a large bowl. Spoon the lentil mixture into the bell peppers, pressing slightly to fill the cavity.
4. Bake the stuffed peppers for 40-45 mins, or until the peppers get tender and the filling is heated through.
5. If desired, serve the stuffed peppers hot, garnished with additional chopped basil.

ROASTED SALMON WITH MANGO SALSA

READY IN ABOUT: 15 MIN

READY IN ABOUT: 15 MIN

SERVINGS: 4

Ingredients

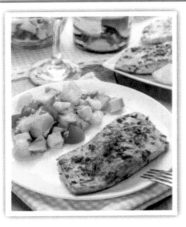

- 4 salmon fillets, 6 ounces each
- Salt and pepper, to taste
- 1 tbsp olive oil
- 1 ripe mango, peeled and diced
- 1/2 cup diced red bell pepper
- 1/4 cup diced red onion
- 1/4 cup chopped fresh cilantro
- Juice of 1 lime
- 1 jalapeno, seeded and minced (optional)

Directions

1. Set the oven to 425°F (220°C) and turn it on. Put parchment paper on a baking sheet.
2. Salt and pepper the salmon fillets and place on the baking sheet. Olive oil the fillets.
3. Prepare the salmon for 12 to 15 mins or until it is fully cooked and can be flaked with a fork.
4. Mango salsa as fish bakes. Mango, red bell pepper, red onion, cilantro, lemon juice, and jalapeño (if using) in a medium bowl. Serve the salmon hot, topped with the mango salsa.

PESTO SPAGHETTI SQUASH WITH CHERRY TOMATOES

READY IN ABOUT: 15 MIN

READY IN ABOUT: 45 MIN

SERVINGS: 4

Ingredients

- 1 medium spaghetti squash
- 1 tbsp olive oil
- Salt and pepper, to taste
- 1 cup cherry tomatoes, halved
- 1/2 cup prepared basil pesto
- 1/4 cup grated Parmesan cheese

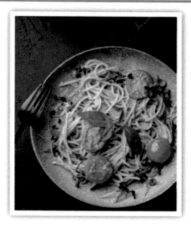

Directions

1. Set up the oven to 400°F (200°C). Prepare parchment paper on a baking pan. Half the spaghetti squash down the middle and take out the seeds. Olive oil and salt and pepper the squash cut sides. Squash cut-side down on the baking pan.
2. Fork-tender squash takes 40–45 minutes to bake. After cooling, use a fork to scrape the squash flesh into spaghetti-like noodles.
3. Mix spaghetti squash, cherry tomatoes, basil pesto, and Parmesan in a large bowl. Serve the spaghetti squash mixture warm with extra Parmesan cheese and fresh basil.

CHICKPEA AND KALE CURRY

READY IN ABOUT: 15 MIN

READY IN ABOUT: 30 MIN

SERVINGS: 4

Ingredients

- 1 tbsp coconut oil
- 1 medium onion, chopped
- 2 cloves garlic, minced
- 1 tbsp grated fresh ginger
- 1 tbsp curry powder
- 1 tsp ground turmeric
- 1/2 tsp ground cumin
- 1/4 tsp cayenne pepper (optional)
- 1 can (14 oz) diced tomatoes
- 1 pack (14 oz) chickpeas, drained and rinsed
- 1 can (14 oz) coconut milk
- 4 cups chopped kale
- Salt and pepper, to taste

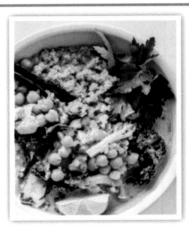

Directions

1. Warm the coconut oil over medium heat in a medium non-stick skillet or Dutch oven. Cook the onion for 5 minutes until tender.
2. Add garlic, ginger, curry powder, turmeric, cumin, and cayenne (if using). Cook for 1-2 minutes or until aromatic.
3. Add diced tomatoes, chickpeas, and coconut milk. Simmer for 20 minutes
4. after boiling. Cook the kale for five minutes or until it has wilted.
5. Salt and pepper the curry to taste. If desirable, serve hot over rice or with naan bread.

BAKED MOROCCAN CHICKEN WITH LEMON AND OLIVES

READY IN ABOUT: 15 MIN

READY IN ABOUT: 45 MIN

SERVINGS: 4

Ingredients

- 4 bone-in, skin-on chicken thighs
- Salt and pepper, to taste
- 1 tbsp olive oil
- 1 small onion, chopped
- 2 cloves garlic, minced
- 1 tbsp ground cumin
- 1 tsp ground paprika
- 1/2 tsp ground cinnamon
- 1/2 tsp ground ginger
- 1/4 tsp cayenne pepper (optional)
- 1 cup chicken broth
- 1 lemon, thinly sliced
- 1/2 cup pitted green olives
- 2 tbsp chopped fresh cilantro

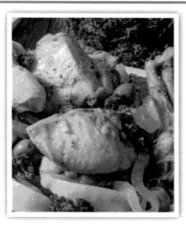

Directions

1. Warm up the oven to 375°F (190°C). Salt and pepper chicken thighs.
2. Heat olive oil on moderate in a large oven-safe skillet. Cook chicken thighs skin-side down for 5 minutes until golden brown. Flip the chicken and cook for 3 minutes. Transfer the chicken to a serving dish.
3. In the same skillet, soften the onion for 5 minutes. Garlic, cumin, paprika, cinnamon, ginger, and cayenne pepper (if used). Cook for 1-2 minutes or until aromatic.
4. Mix in chicken broth, lemon wedges, and green olives. Return the poultry, skin-side up, to the skillet.
5. Bake the skillet for 35-40 minutes, or until the chicken reaches 165°F (74°C). Serve the chicken hot, garnished with chopped cilantro, and drizzled with the pan sauce.

QUINOA STUFFED PORTOBELLO MUSHROOMS

READY IN ABOUT: 15 MIN

READY IN ABOUT: 25 MIN

SERVINGS: 4

Ingredients

- 4 large portobello mushrooms, stems removed
- 1 tbsp olive oil
- Salt and pepper, to taste
- 1 cup cooked quinoa
- 1/2 cup diced red bell pepper
- 1/2 cup crumbled feta cheese
- 1/4 cup chopped fresh parsley
- 1/4 cup chopped walnuts
- 1 clove garlic, minced

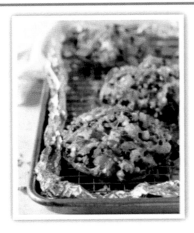

Directions

1. Set the oven's temperature to 375°F (190°C). Line a baking sheet with parchment paper. Place the portobello mushrooms on the prepared baking sheet, gill-side up. Rub the mushrooms with olive oil and season with salt and pepper.
2. Combine the cooked quinoa, red bell pepper, feta cheese, parsley, walnuts, and garlic in a medium bowl.
3. Spoon the quinoa mixture into the portobello mushroom caps, pressing slightly to fill the cavity.
4. Bake the stuffed mushrooms for 20-25 mins or until the mushrooms are soft and the filling is heated thoroughly.
5. Serve the stuffed mushrooms hot, garnished with additional chopped parsley, if desired.

ROASTED BEET AND GOAT CHEESE SALAD

READY IN ABOUT: 15 MIN

READY IN ABOUT: 45 MIN

SERVINGS: 4

Ingredients

- 4 medium beets, scrubbed and trimmed
- 1 tbsp olive oil
- Salt and pepper, to taste
- 6 cups mixed greens
- 1/2 cup crumbled goat cheese
- 1/2 cup chopped walnuts
- 1/4 cup balsamic vinaigrette

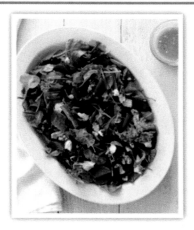

Directions

1. Set the temperature of your oven to 400°F (200°C). Put parchment paper on a baking sheet. Toss the beets with olive oil, salt & pepper on the prepared baking sheet.
2. Fork-tender beets need 45–50 minutes to roast. After cooling, peel and wedge the beets.
3. Mix mixed greens, roasted beet slices, goat cheese, and walnuts in a large bowl. Toss salad with balsamic vinaigrette. Serve salad immediately.

GINGER-GARLIC GLAZED BAKED TOFU

READY IN ABOUT: 15 MIN

READY IN ABOUT: 30 MIN

SERVINGS: 4

Ingredients

- 1 block (14 oz) extra-firm tofu, drained and pressed
- 2 tbsp soy sauce
- 2 tbsp honey
- 1 tbsp rice vinegar
- 1 tbsp grated fresh ginger
- 2 cloves garlic, minced
- 1 tbsp sesame oil
- 1 tbsp cornstarch
- 1 tbsp water
- 2 green onions, chopped
- 1 tbsp sesame seeds

Directions

1. Set your oven's temperature to 400°F (200°C). Prepare parchment paper on a baking pan.
2. On the prepared baking sheet, put 1-inch tofu cubes in a single layer. Soy sauce, honey, rice vinegar, ginger, and garlic in a small pot. Boil it over medium heat.
3. Mix cornstarch and water in a bowl. Cook the cornstarch mixture in the pot for 1-2 minutes until it thickens.
4. Turn off the stove and whisk in the sesame oil while the pan is hot. Pour the sauce over the tofu cubes, turning them to coat all sides.
5. Bake the tofu for 25-30 minutes, turning halfway through, until golden and crispy. Serve the baked tofu hot, garnished with chopped green onions and sesame seeds.

SHRIMP AND ASPARAGUS STIR-FRY

READY IN ABOUT: 15 MIN

READY IN ABOUT: 10 MIN

SERVINGS: 4

Ingredients

- 1 lb large shrimp, peeled and deveined
- Salt and pepper, to taste
- 1 tbsp olive oil
- 1 lb asparagus, trimmed and cut into pieces
- 1/4 cup chicken or vegetable broth
- 3 cloves garlic, minced
- 1 tbsp grated fresh ginger
- 1 tbsp soy sauce
- 1 tsp cornstarch
- 1 tbsp water

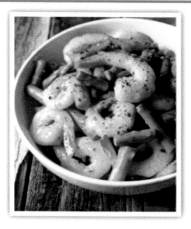

Directions

1. Season the shrimp with salt and pepper. In a medium non-stick skillet or wok, heat olive oil on moderate-high. Cook shrimp for 2-3 minutes until pink and opaque. Move the shrimp to a plate.
2. In the same skillet, sauté asparagus for 4-5 minutes until tender-crisp.
3. Mix broth, garlic, ginger, soy sauce in a small bowl. Put the sauce and asparagus in the pan.
4. Mix cornstarch and water in another small bowl. Cook the cornstarch mixture in the skillet for 1-2 minutes until it thickens.
5. Stir in cooked shrimp. Cook for another 1–2 mins or until everything is hot. Serve the shrimp and asparagus stir-fry hot over rice, if desired.

VEGAN SHEPHERD'S PIE WITH LENTILS

READY IN ABOUT: 20 MIN

READY IN ABOUT: 45 MIN

SERVINGS: 6

Ingredients

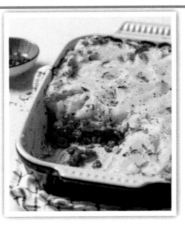

- 2 large sweet potatoes, peeled and chopped
- 1 tbsp olive oil
- 1 medium onion, chopped
- 2 cloves garlic, minced
- 1/2 tsp dried thyme
- 1/2 tsp dried rosemary
- 2 cups cooked green or brown lentils
- 1 cup frozen mixed vegetables (carrots, peas, corn, and green beans)
- 1/4 cup vegetable broth
- Salt and pepper, to taste
- 2 tbsp non-dairy milk (such as almond or soy milk)
- 1 tbsp vegan butter

Directions

1. Set the cooking heat to 375°F (190°C). Grease a 9x13-inch pan. Cook sweet potatoes in boiling water for 15-20 minutes. Drain and reserve.
2. Warm olive oil in a medium skillet on medium. Cook the onion for 5 minutes until tender. Add the garlic, thyme, and rosemary and simmer for one to two minutes or until aromatic.
3. Mix cooked lentils, frozen mixed vegetables, and vegetable broth. Salt & pepper to taste. Cook the vegetables for 5-7 mins or until heated through.
4. Spoon the lentil mixture into the prepared baking dish, spreading it out evenly. In a large bowl, mash the cooked sweet potatoes with non-dairy milk and vegan butter until smooth. Season with salt and pepper to taste.
5. Spread the sweet potato over the lentil mixture in the baking dish, smoothing the top with a spatula.
6. Bake the shepherd's pie for 25-30 mins or until the filling is bubbly and the sweet potato topping is lightly browned. Allow the shepherd's pie to cool for 5 minutes before serving.

WHITE BEAN AND KALE SOUP

READY IN ABOUT: 15 MIN

READY IN ABOUT: 30 MIN

SERVINGS: 6

Ingredients

- 1 tbsp olive oil
- 1 lb lean ground turkey sausage
- 1 medium onion, chopped
- 2 cloves garlic, minced
- 1/2 tsp dried basil
- 1/2 tsp dried oregano
- 6 cups chopped kale, stems removed
- 4 cups low-sodium chicken broth
- 2 (15 oz) cans of white beans (such as cannellini or Great Northern), drained and washed
- Salt and pepper, to taste
- Grated Parmesan cheese for serving (optional)

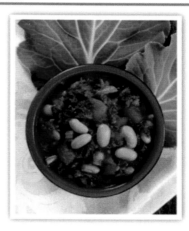

Directions

1. In a large cooking pot, heat the olive oil over moderate heat. Add the turkey sausage and cook, breaking it up with a spoon, until browned and fully cooked.
2. Add the onion to the pot and prepare for 5 minutes or until softened. If using, stir in the garlic, basil, oregano. Cook for 1-2 minutes or until fragrant.
3. Add the kale to the pot and cook, stirring occasionally, for 5 minutes or until wilted.
4. Stir in the chicken broth and white beans, and season with salt & pepper to taste. Take the soup to a boil, then turn down the heat and simmer for 15-20 mins or until the flavors meld.
5. Serve the soup hot, garnished with grated Parmesan cheese, if desired.

EGGPLANT ROLLATINI STUFFED WITH SPINACH AND RICOTTA

READY IN ABOUT: 20 MIN

READY IN ABOUT: 35 MIN

SERVINGS: 4

Ingredients

- 2 medium eggplants, sliced lengthwise into 1/4-inch thick strips
- 2 tbsp olive oil
- Salt and pepper, to taste
- 1 (15 oz) container of ricotta cheese
- 1 large egg, beaten
- 1 cup chopped fresh spinach
- 1/4 cup grated Parmesan cheese
- 1/4 cup shredded mozzarella cheese
- 1/4 tsp ground nutmeg
- 2 cups marinara sauce

Directions

1. Set your oven's temperature to 375°F (190°C). Grease a 9x13-inch baking dish. Rub the eggplant slices with olive oil and season with salt and pepper. Arrange the slices on a baking sheet in a single layer.
2. Bake the eggplant slices for 10-15 minutes or until tender and slightly browned. Take them out of the oven and cool down for a few minutes.
3. Combine the ricotta, egg, spinach, Parmesan, mozzarella, and nutmeg in a medium bowl. Season with salt and pepper to taste.
4. Layer 1 cup of marinara sauce in the baking dish. Place a spoonful of the ricotta mixture at one end of each eggplant slice. Roll up the eggplant slices tightly around the filling and place them seam-side down in the baking dish.
5. Spoon the remaining marinara sauce over the eggplant rollatini. Bake the eggplant rollatini for 20-25 minutes or until heated and bubbly.
6. If desired, serve the eggplant rollatini hot, garnished with additional Parmesan cheese.

CHICKEN FAJITA SALAD WITH AVOCADO DRESSING

READY IN ABOUT: 20 MIN

READY IN ABOUT: 15 MIN

SERVINGS: 4

Ingredients

- 1 lb boneless, skinless breasts of chicken sliced into thin strips
- 1 tbsp olive oil
- 1 tsp chili powder
- 1 tsp ground cumin
- 1/2 tsp smoked paprika
- Salt and pepper, to taste
- 1 red bell pepper, sliced
- 1 yellow bell pepper, sliced
- 1 small red onion, sliced
- 6 cups mixed greens
- 1 avocado, peeled, pitted, and chopped
- 1/4 cup chopped fresh cilantro
- 1/4 cup fresh lime juice
- 1/4 cup plain Greek yogurt without added sugar
- 1 garlic clove, minced
- 1/4 tsp salt

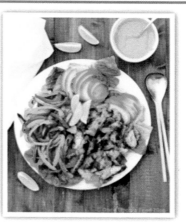

Directions

1. Warm olive oil in a large skillet on medium-high. Cook chicken strips for 5-6 minutes until browned and done.
2. Add chile powder, cumin, smoked paprika, salt, and black pepper to the pan. Stir to season the chicken evenly.
3. Cook the bell peppers and onion in the skillet for 5-7 minutes until tender-crisp. Blend or process avocado, cilantro, lime juice, Greek yogurt, garlic, and salt. Process until creamy and smooth.
4. To serve, divide the mixed greens among four plates. Top each plate with the chicken fajita mixture and drizzle with the avocado dressing.

SWEET POTATO, BLACK BEAN, AND SPINACH ENCHILADAS

READY IN ABOUT: 20 MIN

READY IN ABOUT: 35 MIN

SERVINGS: 4

Ingredients

- 2 medium sweet potatoes, peeled and diced
- 1 tbsp olive oil
- 1 small onion, chopped
- 2 cloves garlic, minced
- 1 (15 oz) pack of black beans, drained and rinsed
- 2 cups fresh spinach, chopped
- Salt and pepper, to taste
- 8 large whole wheat tortillas
- 2 cups enchilada sauce
- 1 cup shredded Monterey Jack

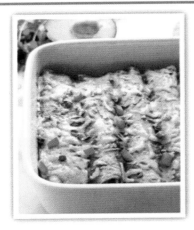

Directions

1. Turn the temperature on the oven to 350°F (180 degrees Celsius). Grease a 9x13-inch pan. Cook sweet potatoes for 10–12 minutes in boiling water. Drain and s tore.
2. Warm olive oil in a large non-stick skillet on medium. Cook the onion for 5 minutes until tender. Cook garlic for 1-2 minutes until aromatic.
3. Mix cooked sweet potatoes, black beans, and spinach. Salt & pepper to taste. Wilt spinach for 3–4 minutes.
4. In the bottom of the baking dish that has been prepared, spread a half cup of the enchilada sauce.
5. Spread sweet potato mixture on tortillas. Wrap the tortillas around the filling and lay them seam-side down in the baking dish.
6. Sprinkle the tortillas with shredded cheese and the remaining enchilada sauce. Bake the enchiladas for 20–25 mins until the cheese is bubbling.
7. Serve the enchiladas while they are still hot, and if you like, garnish them with some additional chopped spinach.

BUTTERNUT SQUASH AND LENTIL COCONUT CURRY

READY IN ABOUT: 15 MIN

READY IN ABOUT: 45 MIN

SERVINGS: 6

Ingredients

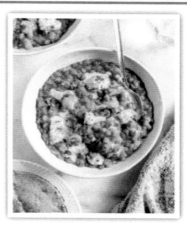

- 1 tbsp coconut oil
- 1 large onion, chopped
- 3 cloves garlic, minced
- 1 tbsp freshly grated ginger
- 2 tbsp curry powder
- 1/2 tsp ground turmeric
- 1/4 tsp cayenne pepper (optional)
- 1 butternut squash, peeled, seeded, and diced
- 1 cup dried green or brown lentils, washed and drained
- 4 cups low-sodium vegetable broth
- 1 (13.5 oz) can full-fat coconut milk
- Salt and pepper, to taste
- 4 cups chopped kale or spinach
- Cooked brown rice for serving
- Fresh cilantro for garnish

Directions

1. Warm the coconut oil in a large non-stick skillet over medium heat. Cook the onion for 5 minutes until tender.
2. Cook garlic and ginger until fragrant, 1-2 minutes. Add curry powder, turmeric, and cayenne pepper (if using) and toast for 1 minute.
3. Butternut squash, lentils, vegetable broth, and coconut milk go in the saucepan. Season to flavor with salt and pepper. Once the curry boils, reduce the heat and simmer for 30–40 minutes until the squash and lentils are cooked.
4. Add kale or spinach and simmer for 5 minutes until wilted. Serve the curry hot over cooked brown rice, garnished with fresh cilantro.

TURKEY AND SPINACH STUFFED BELL PEPPERS

READY IN ABOUT: 20 MIN

READY IN ABOUT: 40 MIN

SERVINGS: 4

Ingredients

- 4 large bell peppers, tops removed and seeded
- 1 lb lean ground turkey
- 1 tbsp olive oil
- 1 small onion, chopped
- 2 cloves garlic, minced
- 1 tsp ground cumin
- 1 tsp dried oregano
- 1/2 tsp smoked paprika
- Salt and pepper, to taste
- 2 cups chopped fresh spinach
- 1 cup cooked quinoa
- 1/2 cup tomato sauce
- 1/4 cup crumbled feta cheese

Directions

1. Set the oven to 375°F (190°C). Coat a 9x13-inch baking dish with oil. Warm oil in a large non-stick skillet on medium-high heat. Add the ground turkey and brown it with a utensil while breaking it up.
2. Simmer the onion for 5 minutes or until it has softened. Cook garlic, cumin, oregano, smoked paprika, salt, and pepper for 1-2 minutes until fragrant.
3. Cook the spinach for three to four minutes or until it has wilted. Remove the skillet from heat and add the cooked quinoa and tomato sauce.
4. Fill bell peppers with turkey mixture and lay upright in the baking dish. Bake for 30 minutes with foil. Uncover the casserole, sprinkle the stuffed peppers with feta cheese, and bake for 10 minutes until the cheese melts and the peppers tender.
5. Serve the stuffed peppers hot, garnished with additional fresh spinach.

SPAGHETTI SQUASH WITH ROASTED RED PEPPER SAUCE

READY IN ABOUT: 15 MIN

READY IN ABOUT: 45 MIN

SERVINGS: 4

Ingredients

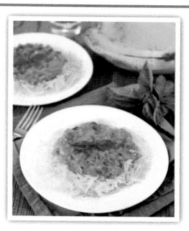

- 1 spaghetti squash, cut in half lengthwise and seeded
- 1 tbsp olive oil
- Salt and pepper, to taste
- 2 cups jarred roasted red peppers, drained
- 1/2 cup raw cashews, soaked in hot water for 15 minutes and drained
- 1/4 cup grated Parmesan cheese
- 2 cloves garlic, minced
- 1 tsp dried basil
- 1/4 tsp red pepper flakes (optional)
- 1/4 cup fresh basil, chopped, for garnish

Directions

1. Set the temperature of your oven to 400°F (200°C). Put parchment paper on a baking sheet.
2. Salt and pepper the cut sides of the spaghetti squash brushed with olive oil. Squash cut-side down on the baking pan.
3. Bake the squash for 40-45 mins or until tender and easily pierced with a fork. Let the squash cool slightly before using a fork to scrape the spaghetti-like strands.
4. While the squash is baking, prepare the roasted red pepper sauce by combining the roasted red peppers, soaked cashews, Parmesan cheese, garlic, dried basil & red pepper flakes (if using) in a blender or food processor. Blend until smooth and creamy.
5. Heat the sauce in a saucepan over medium-low heat until warmed through. To serve, divide the spaghetti squash strands among four plates and top with the roasted red pepper sauce. Garnish with chopped fresh basil.

BAKED EGGPLANT PARMESAN WITH FRESH TOMATO SAUCE

READY IN ABOUT: 20 MIN

READY IN ABOUT: 40 MIN

SERVINGS: 4

Ingredients

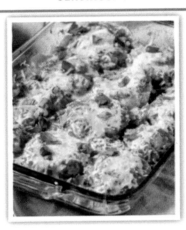

- 2 medium eggplants, sliced into 1/2-inch rounds
- Salt, to taste
- 2 cups fresh whole-grain breadcrumbs
- 1/2 cup grated Parmesan cheese
- 1 tsp dried oregano
- 1 tbsp garlic powder
- 1 tbsp chopped fresh basil
- Freshly ground black pepper, to taste
- 2 large eggs, beaten
- 1 tbsp water
- Olive oil spray
- 2 cups fresh tomato sauce
- 1 cup shredded mozzarella cheese
- Fresh basil for garnish

Directions

1. Set up the oven to 400°F (200°C). Grease a 9x13-inch baking dish and parchment two baking sheets.
2. Place the eggplant segments in a colander, sprinkle them with salt, and allow them to drain for 15 minutes. Rinse and dry eggplant slices. Mix breadcrumbs, Parmesan, oregano, garlic powder, chopped fresh basil, and black pepper in a shallow bowl.
3. Combine the beaten eggs and water with a whisk in another shallow dish. Coat each slice of eggplant with the egg mixture, then press it into the breadcrumbs to coat both sides. Place the coated eggplant slices on the prepared baking sheets.
4. Lightly spray the eggplant slices with olive oil and bake for 15 minutes. Flip the slices and bake for 15 minutes until golden brown and tender.
5. To assemble the eggplant Parmesan, spread 1 cup of fresh tomato sauce in the bottom of the prepared baking dish. Layer half of the baked eggplant slices over the sauce, then top with another cup of sauce and 1/2 cup of shredded mozzarella cheese. Repeat with the remaining eggplant, sauce, and cheese.
6. Bake the eggplant Parmesan for 20-25 minutes or until the cheese is melted and bubbly. Let the dish cool for 5 mins before serving, garnished with fresh basil.

SKILLET RAVIOLI LASAGNA

READY IN ABOUT: 10 MIN

READY IN ABOUT: 25 MIN

SERVINGS: 6

Ingredients

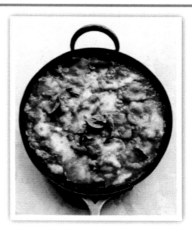

- 1 tbsp olive oil
- 1 small onion, chopped
- 3 cloves garlic, minced
- 1 lb lean ground turkey or beef
- 1/2 tsp dried oregano
- 1/2 tsp dried basil
- Salt and pepper, to taste
- 1 (25 oz) package of frozen cheese gluten-free ravioli
- 2 cups baby spinach, chopped
- 1 1/2 cups shredded mozzarella cheese
- Fresh basil for garnish

Directions

1. Heat olive oil on moderate heat in a large oven-safe skillet. Cook the onion for 5 minutes until tender. Cook garlic for 1 minute until aromatic.
2. Add ground turkey or beef to the skillet and brown, breaking it up with a spoon. Mix in the salt, pepper, oregano, and basil.
3. Turn the oven's temperature to 375°F (190°C). Stir frozen ravioli to coat them.
4. Bring the blending to a simmer, reduce the heat, cover the skillet, and cook for 8-10 minutes until the ravioli is cooked.
5. Cook the chopped spinach by stirring it gently for 2-3 mins or until it softens. Spread the mozzarella over the pasta mixture in an even layer. Bake the skillet for 10-12 minutes until the cheese is bubbling.
6. Take the pan out of your oven and let it cool for 5 minutes. Add some fresh basil to the top.

SHEET-PAN CHICKEN FAJITA BOWLS

READY IN ABOUT: 15 MIN

READY IN ABOUT: 25 MIN

SERVINGS: 4

Ingredients

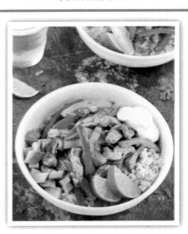

- 1 lb. of boneless, skinless chicken breasts sliced into thin strips
- 3 bell peppers (red, yellow, and green) sliced into thin strips
- 1 large red onion, thinly sliced
- 2 tbsp olive oil
- 1 tbsp chili powder
- 1 tsp ground cumin
- 1 tsp smoked paprika
- 1/2 tsp garlic powder
- Salt and pepper, to taste
- 2 cups cooked brown rice or quinoa
- 1 avocado, sliced
- 1/2 cup cherry tomatoes, halved
- 1/4 cup chopped fresh cilantro
- Lime wedges for serving

Directions

1. Set the oven's heat to 400°F (200°C). Paper-line a large baking sheet. Mix the chicken, bell peppers, and onion in a big bowl.
2. Add olive oil, chili powder, cumin, smoked paprika, garlic powder, salt & pepper in a small bowl. Toss chicken and veggies in a spice mixture.
3. Layer the chicken and vegetables on the baking sheet. Prepare for 20 to 25 mins or until the chicken and veggies are soft.
4. To serve, divide the cooked brown rice or quinoa among four bowls. Top each bowl with the cooked chicken fajita mixture, avocado slices, cherry tomatoes, and chopped cilantro. Serve with lime wedges on the side.

CREAMY MUSHROOM & SPINACH PASTA

READY IN ABOUT: 10 MIN

READY IN ABOUT: 20 MIN

SERVINGS: 4

Ingredients

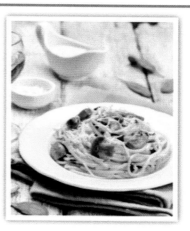

- 8 oz whole wheat pasta (e.g., penne, fusilli, or farfalle)
- 2 tbsp olive oil
- 1 small onion, finely chopped
- 3 cloves garlic, minced
- 8 oz cremini mushrooms, sliced
- 4 cups fresh baby spinach
- 1 cup low-sodium vegetable broth
- 1/2 cup plain Greek yogurt without added sugar
- 1/4 cup grated Parmesan cheese
- Salt and pepper, to taste
- Crushed red pepper flakes, optional, to taste
- Fresh parsley, chopped, for garnish

Directions

1. Cook pasta al dente as per package directions. Drain and store. In a big pan, heat the olive oil over a medium-low flame. Cook the onion for 3-4 mins until it gets softened.
2. Add the garlic and prepare for 1 min or until the garlic smells good. Add in the sliced mushrooms to the pan and prepare for 5 to 6 minutes or until they give off water and soften.
3. Add baby spinach and simmer for 2-3 minutes until wilted. Simmer the skillet with vegetable broth. Reduce for 3-4 minutes.
4. Then add Greek yogurt, Parmesan cheese, salt, and pepper. Add crushed red pepper flakes for spice. Toss cooked pasta with creamy mushroom and spinach sauce in the skillet.
5. Serve the pasta in bowls, garnished with chopped fresh parsley.

CHICKEN & VEGGIE QUESADILLA

READY IN ABOUT: 15 MIN

READY IN ABOUT: 10 MIN

SERVINGS: 4

Ingredients

- 2 cups cooked, shredded chicken breast
- 1 cup bell pepper, thinly sliced (any color)
- 1 cup red onion, thinly sliced
- 1 cup zucchini, thinly sliced
- 1/2 cup corn, fresh or frozen and thawed
- 1 tsp ground cumin
- 1 tsp chili powder
- Salt and pepper, to taste
- 8 whole wheat tortillas
- 1 1/2 cups of shredded cheddar cheese or Mexican blend cheese
- 2 tbsp olive oil, divided
- Sour cream, salsa, and avocado, for serving (optional)

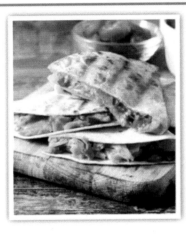

Directions

1. Combine the shredded chicken, bell pepper, red onion, zucchini, and corn in a large bowl. Toss in the cumin, chile powder, salt, and pepper before serving.
2. Spread out four tortillas and divide the cheese equally between them. Cover each tortilla with chicken and veggie mixture. Make a sandwich by gently pressing another tortilla on top.
3. Medium-heat a large non-stick skillet with 1 tablespoon of olive oil. Carefully place one quesadilla in the skillet and cook for 3-4 mins on every side until the cheese gets melted and the tortilla gets a touch of golden brown. Repeat with the remaining quesadillas, adding olive oil to the skillet as needed.
4. Let the quesadillas cool for a minute before cutting each into 4 wedges. If desired, serve the quesadillas with sour cream, salsa, and avocado on the side.

PROSCIUTTO, MOZZARELLA & MELON PLATE

READY IN ABOUT: 15 MIN

READY IN ABOUT: 0 MIN

SERVINGS: 4

Ingredients

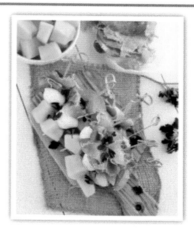

- 8 thin slices prosciutto
- 1 small cantaloupe or honeydew melon, seeds removed and cut into wedges
- 8 oz fresh mozzarella cheese, cut into slices or small balls (bocconcini)
- 2 cups fresh arugula
- 1/4 cup extra-virgin olive oil
- 2 tbsp balsamic vinegar
- Salt and pepper, to taste
- Fresh basil leaves for garnish

Directions

1. Arrange the prosciutto slices, melon wedges, and mozzarella cheese on a large serving platter.
2. Scatter the arugula over the prosciutto, melon, and cheese. In a bowl, whisk together the oil and balsamic vinegar. Season with salt and pepper to taste.
3. Drizzle the dressing over the platter, and garnish with fresh basil leaves. Serve immediately as a light and refreshing dinner option.

Made in the USA
Las Vegas, NV
12 April 2024

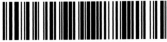